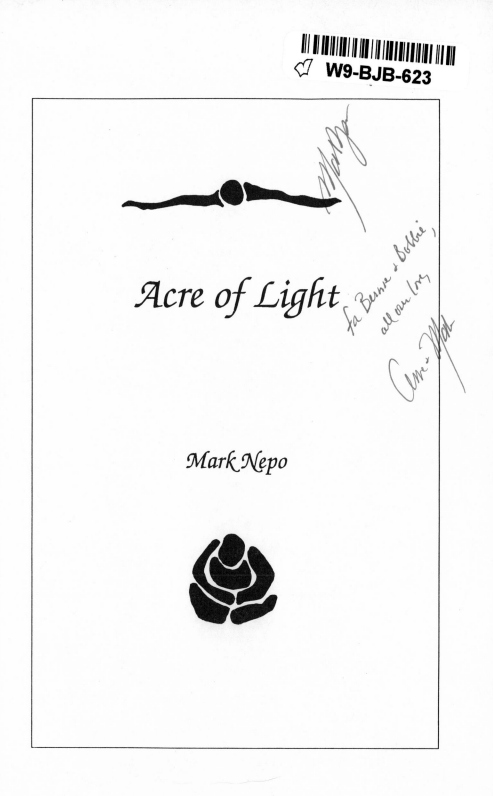

# Acre of Light

## Mark Nepo

Distributed by:
The Talman Co., Inc.
131 Spring St.
New York, NY 10012
(212) 431-7175  Fax (212) 431-7215

*In life one plays the hand one is dealt to the best of one's ability. Those who insist on playing, not the hand they were given, but the one they insist they should have been dealt - these are life's failures. We are not asked if we will play. That is not an option. Play we must. The option is how.*

*-Anthony de Mello*

*for any spirit*
*suddenly awakened*
*to how deep its life*
*how short its stay*

# Preface

*During 1987 my wife and I were both stricken with cancer. The months became a labyrinth. In May Anne was diagnosed as having cervical in situ. This led to her having a conization in June and a hysterectomy that August. At the same time, I had a mysterious lump forming on my head, which turned out to be growing underneath the skull as well. It grew to the size of half a grapefruit. And so, mere days after her surgery, I entered the hospital, moving through a gauntlet of tests, including a biopsy which diagnosed this strange lesion as a lymphoma lodged between my brain and skull. It was eating through the bone. Finally, after much desperation and prayer and visualization and fighting with and against doctors, the tumor, both below the skull and above, vanished, avoiding major brain surgery, whole head radiation and spinal chemotherapy.*

*The doctors could not explain it and our friends and family helped us limp back to life, a struggle in itself, which we were shaping strongly until November of '88 when a spot on my 8th rib began to grow. We were crushed. By January, a lump filled my wife's palm as we hugged. And in February of '89, I underwent thoracic surgery to remove that rib and its adjacent muscles. The cells in that rib had turned more malignant and so, barely repaired, we embarked on four months of chemotherapy. Today, as of our last checkup, we are both well, and forever changed for this odyssey.*

*We have, quite frankly, found death at our shoulder earlier than most. Yet we have also been touched by a relentless, mysterious grace which has surfaced briefly to restore us. Repeatedly, it rises to save us or empower us - we can no longer make the distinction - and we find ourselves tied* to a fathomless place where neither of us had dared to voyage. We call that reservoir God, though you may call it something else.

At first, we thought these poems would bear witness to our struggle, and they do, but they reach beyond the actual moments of trauma and medicine. They have evolved, rather, into a spectrum of how this experience unravelled the way we see the world, how this trauma has scoured our lens of perception. They land, we hope, in a deeper sense of living. And though these pages are written in my voice and in my hand, this book is authored with the blood spilled among us and the spirit that flows between us.

Though our story is framed around a particular crisis, cancer, we believe that crisis of the deepest kind somehow raises a common instinct to survive and with that a common set of tools becomes available to all. And coming this far, it seems clear that being a survivor is embracing the will to live, and whether that embrace lasts for years or months or days or even hours, whoever embraces life **is** a survivor.

Our intent, here, is to be honest with our fears and hopes; to render, through our experience, the irreduceable mystery of life in which we all swim and from which we all emerge to our separate shores. We know we were and are both weak and strong, stubborn and determined, afraid and brave, intrusive and demanding, resilient and stalled, confused and clear - sometimes all at once. We know now that going on without denying any aspect of the human drama is what strength is all about.

-Mark Nepo

# Acre of Light

Preface

It  1
Willfulness  3
The Garage  6
In Voices Half as Loud  9
Tu Fu's Reappearance  13
Without Notice  14
The Waiting Room  15
Knowing God  16
October Storm  17
Inside the Miracle  19
Soft as Satisfaction  21
Living with the Wound  22
God, Self, and Medicine  25
Post-Op  30
Setting Fires in the Rain  32
Mind Sweats  33
Letting Go  35
Surviving has made me Crazy  36
The Decision for Therapy  37
First Treatment  39
Cradlesong  40
Victory with Two Trumpets  42
For Nur  45
Cracked or Healing  47
Love-Sufferings  49
For That  51
Letter Home  54
Endgame 57

Grateful acknowledgment is made to *Voices, the Journal of the American Academy of Psychotherapists,* for first publishing *God, Self, and Medicine,* and our deep thanks to Lars Turin for his gift of *Self,* from which the cover and title page illustrations are taken and newly drawn by the artist himself. And finally, I would like to recognize with love the courageous efforts of my wife, Anne Myers Nepo, who not only lived this, but was instrumental in the editing and thematic design of this book.

# Acre of Light

# It

*First It was a woman with auburn hair*
*whose head would moan when I'd kiss her neck.*
*Then It was a game where despite the others*
*I would rise in the air and toss the ball*
*as if it were all that mattered of me*
*and I'd only feel complete when it*
*slipped the net, touching nothing,*
*just falling blissfully from the sky.*
*Then It was a solitude that overwhelmed*
*me, on a mountain, or lingering by a brook*
*longer than the others. Or talking for hours*
*till the words were strewn like clothes and*
*there was nothing to repeat. And then It was*
*Grandma wearing down to a precious set of bones*
*and I made pilgrimage to hear her secrets once*
*she could no longer speak. And when you went*
*into surgery, I fogged the sliding doors,*
*watching your stretcher grow smaller,*
*believing It was thinning there*
*between us. But now, I am rightfully*
*tired of the chase and It has changed,*
*as have I, from something outside of us*
*we reach for to something that was deep*
*within all along. I've stopped asking*
*for things to emulate, have stopped pushing.*
*Some say I am getting old. Even so, I can't*
*find the words in stream or sky to make clear*
*what I've found. Just stay near long enough*
*and my eyes will tell and we will both*
*let down, unsure what to do next. This*
*is a sign. For It is **here, in us** as*

*we bend. O how this life unfolds, just*
*one concentric womb enroute to another,*
*each encompassing the last; the labor*
*before us, our tunnel to the future;*
*the film covering our eyes, torn*
*away slowly, as we form inwardly,*
*no longer able to pretend.*

# Willfulness
## (for Nur)

To inhale
enough of the world
when you're told
you have cancer
so the dark fruit
never seems larger
than your orbit.

To do what you
have never done
to stay in the
current of life.

To fly 1000 miles
to meet someone
you dreamt
might help.

To pray in tongues
you've dismissed.

To think in ways
others distrust.

To use money
like a shovel
to dig
for time.

*To cross*
*the grasslands*
*between us with*
*a tongue like*
*a machete*
*cleanly*
*sweeping*
*a path.*

*To weep*
*when the pain*
*won't stop.*

*To breathe slowly*
*when the weeping*
*won't stop.*

*To insist*
*that friends*
*don't pamper you*
*or look at you*
*as sentenced*
*or contagious.*

*To slap the thought*
*from their eyes*
*with your heart.*

*To climb the days*
*like mountains*
*for moments*
*like summits*
*where the light*
*spreads your face*

*and the constant
wind makes you forget
the pains in
getting there.*

*To stand as tall
as the weight
you are bearing
will allow.*

*To rely
on your spirit
which waits within
like a thoroughbred
for the heel
of your will
in its ribs.*

*To feel
the vastness
of night
and know
you still
have love
to fill it.*

*To accept
you can snuff
in a gust, but
to stay devoted
to the art
of flicker.*

# The Garage

*-took place while planning for Anne*
*to have her hysterectomy. She was doing*
*her doctoral work in New York that summer*
*and was home only on weekends.*

*That first week away, I thought, with her life so pulled and splintered, I could at least keep our home in order. So often, when things become chaotic and complex, she involves herself in cleaning or fixing or refinishing. But here, there wasn't even time to affect such a sublimation when she needed it most.*

*I sought to surprise her and do something she has asked for years - clean the garage, which had become a quagmire of suburban refuse: tires to cars long gone, copper caps to nothing, buckets with split bottoms, unravelled wicker baskets, fluorescent lamps with no bulbs, cardboard boxes to appliances we can't even find, rusted hibachis, labelless wine and sandpaper worn smooth and O yes, dead mice floating in an open bottle of anti-freeze. It took 14 hours and three trips to the dump and two to the Salvation Army. I was pleased. I had scaled the inept homeowner's Everest. The summit was sparse, swept, labelled, organized, symmetric, emitting a rational if sterile peace.*

*So that first Friday home, after taking her exams, after light wine and soft stories renewed our closeness, I showed her the garage and she began to erupt and suppress, by turns, a semi-hysterical rage. My stomach knotted. I couldn't understand. I tried to explain. She tried to explain. She feared everything she'd ever saved was trashed. I assured her I had exercised conservative judgment. She asked about Paul and*

6

Anne's iron sculpture -- I'd thrown it out. She asked about her parents' lawn chairs -- I'd thrown them out.

She burst into momentary rage, "Someday, I'll clean out **your** belongings!"

I shot back, "How can you talk revenge?! I thought you'd be **pleased!** I busted my ass -"

"I know what you intended and I **do** appreciate it." Then she held her head and walked to the window and broke down, "Can't you understand? I'm losing control over everything in my life. My health. My work. My schooling. My body. And now, I can't even control my home. Can't even have control over my past."

She began to weep uncontrollably.

I felt a gnawing rising tightening twist beneath my ribs. It felt like a burning mix of love and stupidity. I know her so well. How can such care and knowledge blunder, as if I'm always spilling some favorite dish all over her lap. Had she not had her powerless lens on, she would have been pleased.

We worked it through like resilient doves. Neither of us wanted to fight, least of all with each other. I took her to me gently and offered, "I am ready to be anything, anything that will make you feel the peace you deserve."

She held me close. She has moods quick and fragile as a hummingbird. We quivered and held on and repaired.

That night, there was such a quelling safety in sleeping together. We relaxed for the first time in weeks, side by side, each body a wing to the thing between us that believes it can fly. And then to wake with nightwarmth about the neck and throat and chest, to have heads rubbing half-awake in old familiar ways by reflex of a thousand faithful nights - there is no joy, not even the rush of climax, as permeating as the deep habit of

7

*sleeping entangled with an old, old lover.*

*In the morning, unexpectedly, we saw a goldfinch with its small brilliant chest flutter at our window, and Anne told me, her stare fixed on the patch of clearness where the finch had been, that they turn brownish in winter to match the trees and yellow in summer to fool the bees. She is so lovely, my mind cracks like a heartened voice. What must a spirit do to fool disease?*

*We had fruit salad on the deck in the sun and she stared at me in the same soft way I have been falling into her. She finally said in a tone that precedes emotion, "I couldn't imagine myself living with any other man." It was then we realized the robin had hatched her eggs in the maple. Two red twittering beaks jerked up and disappeared, making the most strident and unfinished of moans.*

*Thank God we didn't disturb the nest. Such a simple ingredient to mortality - do not disturb the nest. That's what the garage was all about. Do not disturb the nest. The watering of her flowers has become more symbolic by the day, as if I'm watering her insides, fussing over veins that lean and small organs that curl.*

# In Voices Half as Loud

The MRI bounced its waves across my skull
and there, below, like some magnetized pond,
cerebral fluid pressing on my brain,
the bone worn through. Craneotomy was
on order. I was admitted and pumped with
dilantan to prevent seizures and the hepburn
well was slipped in a vein on my right forearm,
#18, taped and initialled. And the anesthetist
came to interview: had I ever been under? Was I
mildly or moderately aware? Would I call myself
nervous? She said, "Don't be alarmed if you
wake with a tube down your throat.
It's there to help you breathe."

My family came great distances,
unsure what to say. I felt well, alive,
afraid this liturgy would pour the spirit
off my brain. I had dreams of my surgeon
tipping my agitated head like an immature
coconut; he breathing gingerly through his
mask; me hovering above the swollen cannister
that was me. The kind Irish nurse came on her
day off to show my wife where I'd wake, where
they'd stir me to make **sure** I would wake and
dilate and squeeze their well-trained fingers.

We began to pray for a miracle. What had I done?
What could we do? We prayed for a miracle.
To her God, to my God, to anything
more commanding than we. Dear friends
gave us crystals, highly polished with

*their care, and one, a petal from Lipa*
*in the Phillipines where Mary once appeared.*
*They say she loved the air till it rained petals,*
*hours of red from the sky. The petal, in a locket,*
*in a soft gold purse. And we prayed for a miracle,*
*not knowing how to ask. Over and over, till the face*
*on our heart stretched in pain. Give us a miracle*
*and we shall speak of it when the winters are too*
*cold for anyone to care. Give us a safe inexplicable*
*way to drink again from the ordinary days. My head*
*was shampooed and I was told to let nothing*
*pass my lips. Everyone said goodbye*
*and rushed to pick up things that*
*weren't there. The day went gray*
*and those who love me envisioned*
*the side they alone can see.*

*At four, our surgeon, face safe as a globe.*
*They pulled the IV. It bled for a while.*
*There was one more test. The bleeding stopped.*
*One more specialist. He was out of town.*
*They sent us home. I walked right out.*
*We ate with friends and slept at home*
*and woke to familiar noises*
*in the trees. We prayed every night.*
*I continued to feel well, whole, unaffected,*
*confused. The tests were mounting: X-ray, ultrasound,*
*CAT-scan, MRI, bone marrow, tubes and tubes of blood,*
*an angiagram where they snaked the magic thread*
*into my brain, coaxing me to hold still,*
*despite the heat, hold still... A week*

10

went by, and back in, laid out as if sleeping
while a bearded man slid needles in my head, a style
he learned in Sweden, three times, four times, and
shakily, he squirted, smeared and dunked the fluid
from my mind. That night we prayed, the flower
from Lipa on my heart, then on my head. To my God.
To her God. Whatever it will be. Let us heal.
The next day, an open biopsy while awake, peering
at the anesthetist, sitting on her stool with her
plastic valves, asking, "How do you feel?" Beneath
the sterile drapes, "How do you feel?" Their steps
were so soft. How do I feel? What odorless colors
were vapors from my head? I was sent home
with a flowered cap to gauze up my stitches.


The operation has been cancelled. I tell you
I feel fine. They tell me it is cancer and tomorrow
I begin six weeks of radiation, of glancing blows,
five burns a week. The side effects, they say,
are trivial: a sunburn in the ear, along
the roof of mouth, a dizzy sensation perhaps
like losing one's grip. Will it stop me from
hearing as I reach? "You have no choice,"
the oncologist says, "the **treatment**
is the miracle. Without it - Lord! -
The house would fall." He's seen it all,
"You're with us now for life." He holds me
up, "There's months of chemo and checkups
and bloodtests down the line."

*Why can't I forge a faith other than through pain?*
*We change the dressing now each night. O why*
*do roots burn in our Gethsemane?*

*Tonight, in voices half as loud,*
*we think of God as another day*
*and like the Jews spit out into the desert,*
*we hope we can **endure** the miracle*
*as we suffer what we pray.*

# Tu Fu's Reappearance

*-the great Chinese poet Tu Fu(712-770)*
*has appeared to me in dreams*
*as a guide*


Out of the yellow mist
he came again, his Oriental beard
in tow. We were on a healthy shore
and he sat cross-legged in the sand,
scratching delicately with a branch,
his slender head down. I crouched
and put it to him, "How do I block
the fear?" He kept scratching the sand
as if he hadn't heard. I grew angry,
"How do I block the fear?!" He lifted
his head and shrugged,
branch waving above him,
"How does a tree
block the wind?"
With that, he
disappeared.

*Faith is no longer a construct, but some vital tool as urgent as an oar in the ocean or a prayer in the modern world. The radiation therapist who cares but can't look us in the eye glances at his watch and tells us that whole head radiation could erase my memory and render my salivary glands useless, which would mean no more taste and incessant dryness, a ropiness in the mouth... My memory and my mouth are my instruments. They are fingers to a pianist, knees to a quarterback. So what am I to do... Life has changed or rather my position in life... When waiting in the ante-room for surgery, we were all lined up, four or five of us, and one by one the masked angels of this medical underworld were hooking us up. Next to me was a young Black girl, a poor innocent inexperienced being terrified of the needle that would make her sleep. So terrified, she moaned before the needle touched her skin. How I felt her moan. But this was her karma. The needle wouldn't take and they had to try four, five, six times until it settled in a vein. I lay there on my back, my last pouch of innocence torn. Who will suture that? I felt her moan. What on Earth is my karma? What do I fear and need to relinquish so deeply that I am here... I have always needed closure, have always planned the days minutely in advance, but as we struggle, it's clear there will be no closure. There will never be closure again. It makes me wonder if there ever was closure or is it just a fabrication like time, a rope of mind which humans need to get by... Is lack of closure my needle which - because I fear it - must be thrust at me four, five, six times until it settles in my spirit's vein? Is this odyssey the shakedown of all my time-tried ways? I have believed in the sea and now, without notice, I am forced to let go of the dory and push out, out, out...*

*The eyes of animals in paintings surround us and I am forced to confess that in the beginning, I, like most, believed I saw something no one else had seen and that feeling of being another Adam fueled my days and sense of worth. And like most, I ingrew my own version of things: lamenting my lack of brotherhood while secretly exalting that I alone could see.*

*In truth, I was starting to shed all this stuff, but it took getting cancer to shake me so thoroughly, and sitting here in a waiting room at Columbia Presbyterian in a ship-wrecked part of New York, staring straight into this old Hispanic woman's eyes, she into mine - I accept that we all seek the peace of wonder, all wince from the weight of knowing, all speak in a different voice.*

*Suddenly, but cumulatively, like the crest of a long building wave, I know that each being born, inconceivable as it seems, is another Adam or Eve, each of us unique **and** common. Now I understand. It is not my separateness that makes me unique, but the depth of my first hand experience. Clearly, as I look around, the most essential things I sense and feel, we all feel. I meet you there. I believe this acceptance is helping me stay alive.*

*This burdened majestic Hispanic grandmother fighting her tumor looks at me across the waiting room without a word on this sweltering day, the way an old Egyptian slave at one oar must have looked at his younger counterpart three oars down: no pretense, no manners, no needed phrases, but simply with a tired soul that will not look away which says: though this body is chained, these eyes are your eyes and they are forever free.*

# Knowing God

O lone crazed bird
singing in the night-

you sing with your whole body
while the rest of us sleep.

I go to close the window
when my wife touches my arm
and we listen.

You call out
like a saint robbed of words.

Are you blind and trapped
in a vision of sun?

Or do you simply see farther
than the rest of us?

Do you see the light coming?

Do you feel the beads of warmth
forming in the dark?

O what has stirred
that thing in you that sings?

Stir me now.
Sing me clean.

# October Storm

When the most important things in our life happen
we quite often don't know, at the moment, what is going on.
-C.S. Lewis

We wake to an enormous rapping at the side of our house and there, the towering cottonwood whose milkpods dust our path in summer is almost with broken back in supplication to the wind and weight of ten to 12 inches of snow. We have no power. No light. No heat. A symbolism for us we cannot brook for long. No power. No light. No heat. The entire region. Over 170,000 homes. They're talking days.

Not only are we recovering from the latest medical lap, but all our favorite trees lie slain, across the watery snow. We lost our shadblow, those delicate three day a year blossoms. All we can hear is the painful endless creaking of limbs that took 30 or 40 years to ring and grow so that on May first or second or third, with ineffable precision each and every year, a beautiful little net of white could welcome us to spring.

No power. And still we pray, more like John Donne today, with more demand and fury than humility and repose - God, why the shadblow?! This never would have happened except the leaves were still turning, holding on for a week or two. They held firm and kept the snow. They wouldn't let go and down they came. The early storm caught them turning. Had they let go, like every other winter, the bare essential stalks would have slipped the winds. What costly lessons of the age.

How do I become lean and leafless in the midst of surgeons and oncologists? How do I let my illness go like a leaf from my body before the storm? I must let go, the last leap of faith, must give myself over, must not be caught turning brilliant, must not go down with the storm. I must not cling to old inner

17

*leaves, old fears, old dreams. I must not break like autumn trees. A brilliant break is still a break.*

*So, in a world were men go long hard years to school to become cosmetic surgeons, surgeons of appearance, in a world where people pay them to rearrange their features so they can never face who they are; in such a world, my last moat before wholeness is to give up all that I am **not**, no matter how thin what remains.*

*My last leap is in that river of light that is God's and mine, that purity of life-force that makes these sore hips dance till the dance relieves the soreness, that purity of search that makes my sore head swim with colorful visions till the timeless elusive colors ease this old mind's ache.*

*The day the trees fell. We're out trudging in the midst of 60 degree sunshine, brilliant accent on the wreckage: orange maples split at the trunk, long slim elms reaching for the sky snapped in frozen gesture, stubborn oaks wishboned and standing. The day the trees fell. As I await word about another biopsy, Anne refuses to let us be driven from our home. For home, she says, is greater than the storm. She boils soup on the kerosun and puts candles by our heads. And as she rocks my fearful being in her arms, I begin to strip the excess that remains. Fat spirits cannot fly. This is the Tao of letting go.*

18

# Inside the Miracle

*Great knowledge sees all in one.*
*Small knowledge breaks down into the many.*
-Chuang Tzu

*Like the deepest wind, it will move us all and remain unseen. I know this siege is over. We are being rocked into the days. And I know already that just as everyone wanted to blame this illness on their partial understanding of disease: it's in your bones, in your food, in the synthetics of your home, the vinyl of your pontiac, in the emptiness of your life, it's in your protein, in your spinal fluid, in your lack of vitamins, it's in your sexuality, in your stress, in your family, your century, it's in your water, in your air.*

*Just so, already, I can forsee that everyone will claim its disappearance for their partial understanding of wellness: it was Jesus, it was Moses, it was our collective prayers, it was the strength of your mind, it was your visualization, your writing, your goodness returning to you, it was the technology of the day, the medicine of the day, the expertise of your doctors, your change in diet, your change in outlook, your ability to endure, your ability to submit, your ability to take charge, your capacity to accept, it was our love for you, it was your love of life.*

*Just so. It has been our lot since the conception of consciousness to praise what we are and blame what we are not. Yet I have been blessed to have a Catholic priest lay his brooding hands on my Jewish head. I have had a woman I've never met lead a Sufi meditation weekly on my behalf. I have had an artist paint his version of Michelangelo to give me strength. And a poet made a bookmark of sweet grass meant to heal. And I have had deep friends pull crystals from the earth and wash them for me to carry as protection. And yet another has given us a petal from the Phillipines which appeared in a miracle in 1948. And old friends in New Hampshire have designed a cancer-free diet which they are assuming with us. And my brother is insisting that I exercise and consume vast quantitites of vitamin C. And a kind woman who has loved us from afar enrolled us both in the daily prayers of yet another religious order in Massachusetts. And a sweet friend who does not believe in God sits with me in silence when I have nothing left to say. And still another dear soul is praying to her dead mother and to Thomas Merton that we be healed. And I even talk to Grandma sometimes or visualize in her golden chairs.*

*Just so. I am blessed that all these efforts carry me. For each is indispensable. Just so. I need Catholic, Jew, Mystic, Sweet Grass, Sufi, Herbs, Crystal, Dead Mother, Dead Grandmother, Dead Monk and Golden Chairs to heal.*

*I only know that everything has helped and I am not great enough or wise enough to break down into percentages how much vitamin, how much medicine, how much prayer, how much God, how much Jesus, and how much mental fight. I only know that those who suffer partial belief are only partially healed.*

# Soft as Satisfaction

*We often pray God will let us have truth.*
*It is more important to pray God will help us live with it.*
*-Robert Penn Warren*

*I was so solid when our lives were crumbling.*
*Why am I powder when you and the days*
*are sturdy as gold?*

*I am fading into ordinary ways: mere scratch*
*of belly, long itch of eyes.*

*I knew all through it, if all else failed,*
*my compassion for the whole like an atom of nectar*
*would fight off death and bring us back.*

*But now, the days seem unmagnified*
*without emergency. Why can't I be brave*
*when mere silence is at stake?*

*I have been fighting the passage*
*into normal life the way a salmon,*
*hooked and set free, tires*
*and starts to slip downstream.*

*Names and praise no longer feed.*
*But more, what scares*
*is the lack of hunger.*

# Living with the Wound

It is not an all or nothing
proposition: be without pain,
without cut or be defeated;
be among the happy
or the broken; to drown
in the world's sadness
or to turn from death
in a gaiety that is
pure denial.

There is a need to be specific
if we are to survive.
It requires being honest,
the way seeing requires
the eyes to stay open.

It means I can tell you
when you hurt me
and still count on your love.

It means being honest
with myself, knowing
the ugly things are not
always someone else's.

The thing that keeps me
from sleeping is a loneliness
that returns no matter
what I learn. One can
only conclude that knowledge
is a dark horse that wants
to throw its rider.

*We only let events in so far,*
*as if the glass-thinking*
*that protects us will shatter*
*if we let things like anger*
*and sadness shout.*

*Practical people cut the cord*
*to those who've broken hope,*
*the way riders shoot horses*
*with broken legs, as if*
*there's nothing to be done.*

*Now I know they do this*
*for themselves, not wanting*
*to care for a horse that cannot run,*
*not wanting to sit with a friend*
*who can't find tomorrow, not wanting*
*to be saddled with anything*
*that will slow them down.*

*The people I know well*
*are always in struggle.*
*"Nice to know losers,"*
*a voice shouts in a bar.*

*But this is the rub of being real:*
*if there is no hill, there is no wheel.*

*I used to think it bad timing.*
*When I was up, you were down.*
*When you were ready,*
*I was scared. But since*
*we've never given up on each other,*
*it's clear that drinking wonder*

*when we're sad is how we shed*
*the grip of being pained.*

*I have a right to joy*
*even when lonely,*
*even when bleeding,*
*and you need never*
*cover your wounds*
*when entering my house.*

*If your voice breaks, I'll be a cup.*
*If your heart sweats, I'll be a pillow*
*in which you'll chance to dream*
*that weeping is singing*
*through an instrument*
*that's hard to reach,*
*though it lands us like lightning*
*in the grasp of each other*
*where giving is a mirror*
*of all we cannot teach.*

# God, Self, and Medicine

*Okakura Kakuzo, the astute Japanese historian, said, "It is in us that God meets with Nature." We are the crucible, the ever-changing inlet through which the greater whole in all its forms ebbs and flows. And everytime the Universe, through Nature or God, flows through us, we are rinsed larger, cleansed and charged yet again. And what is medicine, if not the laws of nature applied to cleanse the self. And what is God, if not the laws of spirit applied to enlarge the self. It implies that to enlarge is cleansing; to grow, healing. Thus, to talk about the art of healing is to investigate the various ways, both natural and spiritual, that the whole, if taken in, can preserve the part.*

*I have a rare form of cancer, and I have learned through this ordeal that my state of well-being fluctuates; in fact, has its own wave pattern: swelling, cresting, crashing. And I have learned that the active presence of these elements - God, Self, and Medicine - affects whether I am cresting or crashing. Moreover, the apparent discord or harmony between these elements has a direct impact on my wholeness at any given time.*

*Initially, I felt a traumatic paralysis, the fast-breathing, huddled fear of a wounded animal lying still in the brush, expecting to be struck again. This is worse than discord, this is withdrawal from anything that can help. This is the power of fear - to make you recoil from anything larger. While in this state, nothing flows through, and therefore, nothing cleanses or enlarges. The part remains cut off when it needs to be connected more than ever. And I believe how we first stand after doubling over is crucial to whether we will heal at all.*

*One is always **thrust** into the world of cancer and there is no escort. When my wife and I were so thrust, we uncannily* *met our counterparts, Janice and Tom. Janice was a strong, determined woman who believed primarily in self. She did not believe in medicine and therefore put her entire well-being and treatment into her own hands. She rejected all medical intervention, and if she utilized anything greater than her self, it remained a secret liaison till the end. She was tenacious but died a painfully drawn out death. And there isn't a doctor's visit I don't feel Janice over my shoulder. I understand her resistance more and more, for the things we're asked to do to preserve our well-being are not pleasant. Yet in the hard breath before each decision, I see her reliance solely on self and fear its imbalance.*

*Tom, on the other hand, was adrift. He really had no sense of self and had a disinterested entropic view of the world. He put his fate completely in the judgment of medicine. And so, we watched Tom grow smaller in the space he took up. We watched Tom give no resistance whatsoever to what doctors wanted to do. Blake said, "Without contraries there is no progression." Tom presented no healthy contrary and thus there was no progression. He became invisible, vanishing piece by piece. By Christmas of that year, he no longer knew who we were. By February, he died.*

*I feel roughly blessed to have Tom and Janice as specters of where I must not go, though the further we travel here, the more compassion I have for how easily, in any given moment, the Tom in me or the Janice in me can take over. But life has become a process wherein God is the undefinable sum and source, despite our moods, from which self and medicine flow. It's as though self and medicine are dancers, exchanging foreground and background; one holds while the other leaps; and always the ground they dance, from which they rise, is God.*

26

*Indeed, medicine is preservation from without, and God is preservation from within. And as the self carves its path of outer treatment, the spirit steers its channel of inner treatment; outer treatment, pathbreaking on land; inner treatment, pathbreaking by sea. We have come to believe that both must be kept active in order to stay well. The self must evolve amphibiously, must walk on land, but retreat to the sea. And though certain rules apply in the jungle, we can never forget that different laws rule the deep.*

*I am drawn to Avicenna's* Poem On Medicine, *the medieval practice manual used in Eastern and Western medical schools for almost 600 years. Though Avicenna remarks on conditions with unusual physical detail, I read them now, a thousand years later, as a citizen of modern oncology, and can't help but take them inwardly, as symptoms of our alignment with the whole.*

*He speaks of messenger signs of death based on actions of the patient: "dimunition in the opening of the eye, deviation of gaze, and fear of light." Our openness is our lifeline. Our vision, our blood. When we begin to close, we turn blue. When we shut the eye or squint on purpose, we lose the courage which looking into things brings. And if we ever fear the light, we are doomed. He speaks of fatal signs: "groping of the hands about the pillow, and if, at the end of sleep, one sees himself covered with snow."*

*I fear these things, for I have groped my pillow, but refuse the snow, and none of it has stayed with me, though each has skirted my being in darker moments. But I believe deeply that openness on the way **out** is as crucial as on the way **in.** For God and Nature **meet** in us. They do not **reside** in us. And I fear that the predominant cause of illness, spiritually, stems from the lodging of what's dark, from the stoppage of that natural* *flow. When we break from the whole, we clog and weaken.*

*As it is, we crest and crash repeatedly. When crashing, the array of negative responses is natural - the specter of recurrence, the tide and rise of mortality into one's thinking, the anticipation that small sores will be called tumors, that sweating, though it is August, might be a symptom - but you can't make a home for it. You must allow it, feel it, and let it pass through. For if you make a home, it will enter and take over your life. You will invite a self-fulfilling prophecy. That's how this works. It bites and waits to see if you'll scratch a hole in which it can stake its claim and fester and spread; physically, emotionally, psychologically. So, it's a constant battle, a constant log-roll - you standing on your woe - first one way, then the other. You must let the range of fears and sorrows through, for to bar them will strangely give them the power to overcome you when you finally let down. So, you can't keep them out, the fears, but you can't let them hover. You must let them, like a muddy stream, enter and flow on through, churning up your bottom, keeping you fresh.*

*Likewise, miracle is a process and not an event, and it yields an inexplicable flood of Universe, surfacing as a sudden untempered restorative; returning the ailing part, the single life, to the healthy whole, the world. Miracle, the logic-defying process by which we churn God, Self, and Medicine into the cream of our consciousness. I think, more often than not, the will brings the self in line with the currents of the whole and healing is the rejoining that takes place; like a dam thrust open for fish to turn and ride the stream. What is self-induced is that inner alignment with the elements which, in turn, yields the deep miracle of health. And if, as Solzhenitsyn suggests, a clear conscience is necessary to induce new growth, it's because the clarity of one's character makes a*

28

*clean funnel of the soul.*

*Avicenna also speaks of the messenger signs of healing,
which I again take inwardly: "when a balanced warmth
appears; when the senses grow acute; when one's movements
take on strength; if one is quiet after a sleep which dissipates
his pain; if a regular respiration appears, neither rapid nor
slow; if the pulse is not restrained but full; and when the
breath of a patient is not burning." This all affirms the laws of
spirit which enlarge the self. And I can attest to these
moments aglow upon which my quest for health is built, no
matter how often I lodge the dark or break from the whole.*

*It seems to me, from this stark vantage point, that to allow
the elements their flow is the only way to health. And to do
that, we must somehow sustain the courage to stay open, to
embrace and let go, to internalize and cleanse, to let fear
decompose within into peace, to let the fear of light expand into
a balanced warmth.*

*Next week, I must lie down in a tethered sleep while they
scrape tissue from my bones again. No one knows where that
will lead. And, of course, I am afraid, but in making this
decision, I heard Janice spurn my doctor and saw Tom with
indifference bow. I believe in God and in this strange familiar
terrain, called me, in which life and He meet. So, I waited till
these elements merged, way down beneath my understanding,
and there, in what felt like calm balance, I said yes, help me.*

# Post-Op

I could see it in your eye
when you thought I was dozing.
You thought you might lose me
and you started to remove yourself
as we do when pets are about to die
or old friends have decided to move.

But we are **living** with this,
not dying from it, and I
am not going, not until
the red bird flies
into the sun.

And you must not
corrupt the time we have
by double-living
what we will not.

So come on back.
Tell me your pain.
Utter your fear.
I feel it anyway.

This I've learned, the pain
makes the secrets known.

And so I saw you
sinking at the foot of my bed
watching the tubes run in
and out, saw you start
to fix the scene in your
future as a sad memory

*of when I went away.*

*Come back to me. Now.*
*There are many futures*
*and each depends on us*
*today.*

*This is not about dying.*
*I have agreed to suffer*
*and therefore will live*
*like a gypsy exhausted*
*from his dance.*

*And you have chosen to love me.*
*So you will play my tambourine.*
*You will coax me to try*
*and urge me to stop.*

*And you will not have me*
*cleanly: in your life or not.*

*No. You will suffer too,*
*as I flare and fade*
*a hundred times,*
*while you marvel*
*at the secrets*
*I cough up from*
*the other side.*

*You see. It was time. The tube had to come out. It had drained my lung of blood for days, through a slit in my side. The doctor was waiting and I looked to Paul at the foot of my bed. Without a word, he knew. All the talk of life was now in the steps between us. He made his way past the curtain. Our arms locked and he crossed over, no longer watching. He was **part** of the trauma and everything - the bedrail, the tube, my face, his face, the curve of blanket rubbing the tube, the doctor pulling the tube's length as I held onto Paul - everything pulsed. And since, I've learned, if you want to create anything - peace of mind, a child, a painting of running water, a simple tier of lilies - you must crossover and hold. You must sweep past the curtain, no matter how clear. You must drop all reservations like magazines in waiting rooms. You must swallow your heart, leap across and join.*

# Mind Sweats

As if it were a secret
we didn't know we were keeping,
a whispered knowledge tucked in the heart
like an envelope with special instructions -
open only if death seems imminent:

our grasp on life
falls apart repeatedly, reassembles repeatedly
like the hold a throated river has on its debris;
as if to follow someone with more confidence
would make a difference.

Thank you for holding me in the night.
It's just at unexpected times the silence
seeps in like water soaking through.
When I am well, this is exciting,
a form of waking naked in the world.
But last night, I felt dispensable.

The mind, at times, can be rubbed
to a blister till this clear fluid
collects and the head grows sore.

In my fright, I know I am going to die.
Not now, not soon, but **know,** the way
seeing all those images on the news,
one finally catches in your throat,
and you **know** that somewhere it is real,
somewhere there is only air between
the camera and the pain.

*Last night, I knew there was only air.*
*And you held me in the dark.*

*We huddle in our love*
*as in a tent on a shore*
*watching our fears roll in like surf -*
*building, crashing, thinning -*
*knowing the swimmer*
*who withstands the pounding*
*can make it past the breakers.*

## Letting Go

*After feeling driven my whole life*
*something very near the center has*
*unwound and I can no longer hurry*
*through airports or return all my calls.*

*And sometimes people I barely know*
*swim up like old worn fish and show me*
*the map of their gills, show me the one long*
*gash of something they once swallowed, show me*
*how it has cut each breath since. And I am*
*honored to warm them like a blanket.*
*But when alone, I find it hard*
*not to watch what I swallow.*

*When alone, these things*
*I've wanted to know since birth*
*feel so unanswerable, I must*
*have been torn from them.*

*I'm sure the hawk doesn't know it's a hawk,*
*anymore than the spirit knows it's being*
*spiritual. Or a screendoor slapping,*
*like a tired life, in the night,*
*if it's opening or closing.*

*Though we give up the murky fears,*
*we still can't know our worth,*
*no more than a faceless treasure*
*can fathom why*
*it was boxed*
*or buried*
*or saved.*

# Surviving has made me Crazy

I eat flowers now and birds follow me.
I open myself like an inlet
and dolphin-like energies
swim on through.

Wherever I go, I remain silent
and the silence begins to glow
till one eye in the light
outsees two in the dark.

When asked, I now hesitate,
for there are so many ways
to love the earth.

I water things now constantly:
water the hearts of dead friends with light,
the sores of the living with anything warm,
water the skies with a thousand affections
and follow the voices of animals
into grasses that move like ocean.

I eat flowers now and birds come.
I eat care and things to love arrive.
I eat time and as I age
whatever I swallow grows timeless.

I eat and undie
and water my doubts
with silence
and birds come.

## The Decision for Therapy

*As we gamble on the future,*
*let's stay clear: this moment*
*with all its promise is intact.*
*It is not up for grabs.*

*This moment for which I've*
*lived all others, for which*
*I've withstood the breakage*
*of all I know repeatedly,*
*this moment is germ-free*
*and not on trial.*

*You are welcome here*
*by permission only*
*and the alarm you cast*
*like a blind fisherman*
*will only snag my want*
*for tomorrow, only hook*
*what I do not have.*

*I know you mean to help*
*and I cannot deny*
*you are a bridge*
*I have to cross.*

*But where I live*
*cannot be staged*
*or stained or seen*
*as gross evidence.*

*Where I live*
*is impervious*
*to histology.*

*It is the one site*
*in the city that*
*will not burn.*

*And if you guide me*
*to tomorrow, I'll*
*show you, as you*
*shake your head,*
*how I still glow*
*in this unbreachable*
*clearing I carry with me*
*like a sun or rising star*
*protected by its rays.*

## First Treatment

We cried in the car last night.
I vowed never to give up, while Anne,
in a moment that made us feel eighty,
said, "If it gets too much, you can."

How much is enough?
How much scouring before the face
wears down its features;
the mind, its beliefs?

How many times can a heart
be made over like the handle of a tool?

When I look into the eyes of those
who love me and not their minds,
when I wash my hands and rinse
my head, when I hear my God
inbetween my suffering,
I realize the gift
like a chisel or harp
is in my hand,
and that you give back
by making good use
of what you're given.

# Cradlesong
## (for Jessica)

How do I explain chemotherapy
to a six year old up in my arms
before I shed my coat?

How do I tell her I can't
kiss her on the lips because
my white count is low, that
we must leave early because
Aunt Helen has a cold?

And when we go, she hides
in her room, face in the corner,
till I return and swallow her
in my arms - Damn it all -
I kiss her anyway
again and again.

And next time, she's on my lap
staring in my eyes as if to see -
is there laughter behind them
or is that puppy on a leash, too?

She searches my face, then says,
"You're losing your hair."

I act surprised, "Where? Show me."
She runs her hand along my scalp.

I lean into her little face,
"It's still me."

*She takes my hand and out we go*
*as she shimmies on her swing,*
*pumping higher, giddy as she*
*eats the day, "Look! Uncle Mark!*
*I'm swinging till I'm High*
*as the Sun! Look!"*

*I push her with all my heart,*
*"Me, too, sweetheart -"*
*she comes back to me -*
*"me, too."*

# Victory with Two Trumpets

*I am tired of those*
*who swill their head*
*in a bucket and claim*
*there is no God or Good*
*or Beauty to be had.*

*I come from a tribe*
*of survivors who love life*
*more than the hardships*
*they've been dealt. And*
*we have found each other*
*the way rivers find the sea.*

*We know pain and struggle*
*and fear like driftwood*
*and glass scraping at*
*our bottom. But have*
*grown love and faith*
*and will like barnacles,*
*razored out of sight.*

*We come from every sort*
*of rock: drunken, raped,*
*abandoned, cancered.*

*And though everyone*
*navigates their darker*
*moments, though everyone*
*trembles at the wheel,*
*each is strong, that is real,*
*working naked in the stream.*

*So I am fed up with those*
*who suck at the dark side*
*of things, complaining*
*they are bored, complaining*
*life's a chore, complaining*
*there is nothing but their*
*chaos to applaud.*

*To be broken is no reason*
*to see all things as broken.*

*To fear death*
*is not a calling.*

*I have outlived a tumor*
*pressing on my brain, have*
*had my 8th rib removed, and*
*though I wept in the tub*
*at the gash in my side,*
*at the fact that I can*
*be slit open so easily*
*like a bull pumped up*
*for market, I only*
*want life more,*
*long to dance*
*till my heart*
*sweats, till*
*my mind stops*
*anticipating,*
*till I understand*
*the dead tree's part*
*in the design.*

*I long like a root*
*deeper in the earth*
*so I can reach*
*farther to the sky.*

*So don't tell me*
*there's nothing*
*in your bucket.*

*To brush my teeth*
*has significance*
*after three weeks*
*of lying flat. And*
*there's glory*
*in the water*
*from my mouth*
*as it swirls*
*down the sink*
*in rhythm with*
*the largest falls*
*I've never seen.*

*And when the ribs*
*ache, I dream of*
*swimming naked*
*in life's waters*
*with those who*
*pulled me back*
*to this season*
*of mystery*
*so many*
*refuse.*

# For Nur

*I've been terribly busy since you died,*
*fingering my list of things to do*
*like a rosary, veiled in a shroud of activity,*
*afraid to let it in, afraid your death*
*means I am dying too,*
*and when that's passed,*
*sad to think I might*
*go on undaunted*
*without you.*

*After months of furious doing,*
*of painting and planting,*
*after mornings of pondering*
*ancient philosophy,*
*I had my own checkup*
*and in brief moments*
*feared I was you, but*
*as the CAT-scan whirred,*
*I knew I was well*
*and strangely let you go,*
*your presence drifting*
*on its own in the sea*
*that holds us both.*

*Now your father calls.*
*He's packing up your things*
*and says you wanted us to choose*
*something you held close,*
*but each of us will sigh,*
*it was me, as we rummage*
*through your things*

*the way orphans comb*
*the ashes of the past.*

*You were always well,*
*deeply well, no matter*
*the condition of your skin.*

*This morning the busyness is gone*
*and I watch the wind move through*
*the oak, all its leaves astir.*

*Everything seems closer,*
*renewed, and the part of you*
*where I held on has fused*
*these months in the dry way*
*that stubborn souls*
*graft to what's forgiving*
*like broken bones*
*growing white*
*across their break.*

# Cracked or Healing

On the other side, everything,
from the quick song of birds
to the peace trapped within
a fresh brook's gurgle,
everything is rare
and uncertain.

Now I want to stand naked
before every wind, though
I'm frightened I will break.

And all the warrior selves
stand guard, well-trained
for the next crisis: the fingers
search the glands during winter colds,
the eyes trace scars for irregularities,
the heart tightens like a lip
when entering a hospital,
the unfelt part of my journey
cries like a babe
wanting its strange milk
when seeing needles
hang from brittle arms.

But underneath, the oyster
that surrounds my soul
lives like a Queen dethroned
and exiled for her softness,
yet everything that matters
seeps into her cell.

*I wait for her to send the guards*
*away, but with a sort of pity*
*she lets them occupy their time.*
*What else would they do?*

*I have given up the world*
*through her. It peels*
*like a crusted shell.*

*Through her*
*I imitate the moon,*
*lighting the night*
*with reflections*
*of my craters.*

*Survival is the standing watch.*
*But living now is blessing every crack*
*as an opening, treasuring the song*
*that whistles through as God, praying*
*the break to let Him in*
*won't end it all.*

# Love-Sufferings

When I began writing poetry, I almost studied with a tough fiber of a man, Paul Blackburn, but he died of cancer. It shook us all. Later, I read how he regarded his plight, "I want no pity for a pain I would share with no man." I was disturbed. I didn't understand. But now, after having tread my own yard of hell, I still don't understand. Pity is to love what sarcasm is to honest speech, but sharing pain is the only way to stay alive. I am sorry he felt so all alone.

Perhaps when we almost die, we empty our pockets too fast and perhaps too late, but there is no shame in empty pockets or empty moods. And while needing love to feel good about being alive is a modern indulgence, needing love to stay alive is the archetype behind God almost touching Adam's finger. Perhaps, in the original sense of seance, death can be put off, if we simply join our love in earnest expectation that we be touched from the beyond.

I have never wasted my gift. Now, I've had to fight for it. I still am. But not alone. Rather with a net of love which helps absorb and distribute the struggle. It's taught me that if we share pain, which is a lot to ask, there is no room for pity. For the sharing of the struggle requires an investment, a real life-changing investment by those who care; an involvement which will instigate their own tandem suffering. Pity is a bleecher activity. It is the substitute for front line caring.

We are well today, because those who love us got involved, deeply involved, daily involved. And by being so healed, we are forever wed to their pain. We are forever open to their struggles. By being so loved, we can never shut our lives completely again. If they fall, we will live lower. If they rise, we will take on their dizziness. We will live like pools of water; each clearly individual but all sharing and exchanging the

49

*same slippage and rush of tides. Now I understand. This is the basis of human family, the sharing of pain, the investment of love by which we make a difference and are changed, again and again.*

*I have said throughout this ordeal, repeatedly, "Feel bad if you want, but don't feel bad for me or for yourself." It was an instinctual retort which I really didn't understand. But now I understand that touch is the clearest way to know another's experience. To walk through the surf makes us part of the ocean. To watch it swell and recede makes us just a shiftless though sympathetic dune. We are well because people didn't watch our suffering, but entered us and then they felt love-sufferings of their own; which, at times, hurt them too much; which, in turn, forced us to nurture them, until, in bare, essential ways on certain days, we weren't sure who was ill and who was well. A solution that saved us all.*

# For That

*How could I know*
*creating and surviving*
*were so close*

*a membrane apart,*
*a pulsing, glowing film*

*of will, the muscle;*
*faith, the will*
*flexed.*

*How could I know*
*each day*
*is*
*the last*
*and*
*the first*

*and beneath*
*that tension,*
*if we wade below it*
*like the surface*
*of a sea, a chance*
*only coral*
*can feel*

*and there*
*we grow*
*so thoroughly*
*that breaking*
*and healing,*

*creating*
*and surviving,*
*first and*
*last are*
*one, the*
*same.*

*There,*
*beneath*
*the tensions*
*of psychology,*
*beneath the*
*pockets of doubt,*
*beneath the*
*prospect of*
*days to be lived*
*or not lived,*

*a moment*
*so calm*

*it is*
*cleansing*

*and I smile*
*through my*
*whole body*
*just to have*
*a body,*
*just to have*
*this orchestra*
*within that plays*
*to no conductor.*

*Will you believe me then,*
*that like the zen monk*
*who finds wisdom*
*in his fears,*
*who hears more*
*than he can say,*

*will you believe me*
*that no matter what*
*is shucked or diagnosed*
*or bled, I would*
*trade places*
*with no one,*
*spirits*
*with all.*

*My purpose,*
*at last,*
*to hold*
*nothing*
*back.*

*My goal:*
*to live*
*a thousand years,*
*not in succession,*
*but in every*
*breath.*

# Letter Home

You ask if anything's changed.
I write this in an open boat
in the middle of a lake
which has been drawing me
to its secret for months.
I am becoming more like water
by the day. The slightest brace
of wind stirs me through.
I am more alive than ever.
What does that mean?
That in the beginning
I was awakened
as if a step behind,
always catching up,
as if waking in the middle
of some race that started
before I arrived, waking
to all these frantic strangers
hurrying me on,
as if landing in the middle
of some festival not knowing
what to celebrate, as if
someone genuine and beautiful
had offered to love me
just before I could hear
and now I must find her.
You ask if anything's changed.
I am drifting in the lake
and now it's a matter of slowing
so as not to pass it by.

You say I don't sound the same.
It's 'cause I think more like a fish
and only surface to eat.
I used to complain so much,
annoyed that every chore
would need to be done again,
that the grass would grow back
as soon as I'd cut it. Now
I am in awe how it will grow
no matter what you do to it.
How I need that knowledge.
You say I don't try as much with you.
It's 'cause you still behave
as if life is everywhere
but where you are
and I need new knowledge.

It has not all been pleasant.
One of us died the other day.
The last time I saw him,
we held hands through a park fence -
he was thin - but we held on as if
the fence weren't there and as if
he were already on the other side.
Now we pray for him anyway, imagining
peace a lighter affair once gone
like pebbles sinking softly underwater.
I put my palm on the water's surface
lightly, not trying to hold any of it,
just feeling it push back.
You ask and I hesitate.
It seems everything has changed
when, in fact, it is only me.

*I was closed so long, I thought*
*opening was breaking and in rare*
*broken moments I've seen now*
*how your secret is my secret*
*just swallowed at a different time*
*about a different face*
*with a different though equally*
*private name that brings it back,*
*too keenly, too deeply.*

*I write this in an open boat*
*where yards from me the heron*
*perched on turtle rock is spreading*
*its wings in the sun, holding*
*perfectly open and still,*
*the light filling, glazing its eye.*
*I am drifting here, heart spreading*
*like a heron's wing, more alive*
*than I thought possible.*
*You think me indifferent.*
*I want this for you*
*more than you can dream.*
*I am here. Drifting.*
*Come. Please. Swim.*
*If you can.*

# Endgame

Death pushed me to the edge.
Nowhere to back off. And
to the shame of my fears,
I danced with abandon
in his face. I never
danced as free.

And Death backed off,
the way dark backs off
a sudden burst of flame.
Now there's nothing left
but to keep dancing.

It is the way
I would have chosen
had I been born
three times
as brave.

**Mark Nepo** is a poet and philosopher. He earned his Bachelor's degree from SUNY Cortland(1973), and his Doctorate from SUNY Albany(1980), where he continues to teach poetry and creative writing. His books include *God, the Maker of the Bed, and the Painter*(Greenfield Review Press, 1988), and *Fire Without Witness*(British American, Ltd., 1988). He has recently completed two books of spiritual philosophy, *Rowing at the Pace of Clouds* and *While We are Blossoms: the Journey beyond Selfing*. His essays regularly appear in *Voices, the Journal of the American Academy of Psychotherapists* and *Pilgrimage, the Journal of Psychotherapy and Personal Exploration*.